Property of

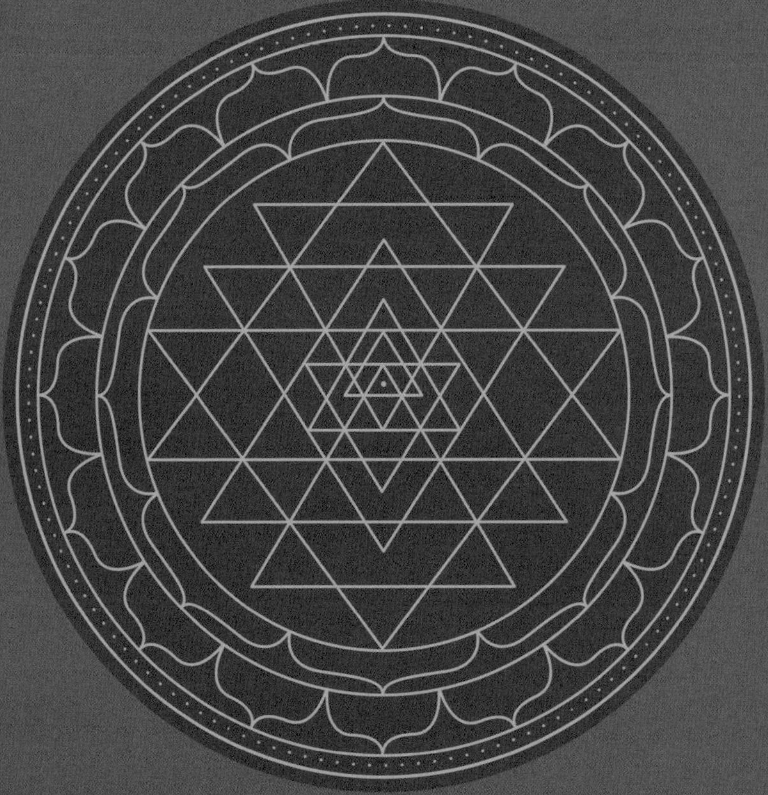

INSIGHTS
A Mandala Journal

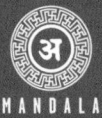

www.mandalaearth.com
Tag us on Instagram! @mandalaearth

Copyright © 2020 Mandala Publishing. All rights reserved.
MANUFACTURED IN TURKEY
10 9 8 7 6 5 4 3 2 1